Essential Oils & Aromatherapy 101

Top Beauty Secrets for Your Health

By Katie Lenhart
Copyright © 2013

Income Disclaimer

This book contains business strategies, marketing methods and other business advice that, regardless of my own results and experience, may not produce the same results (or any results) for you. I make absolutely no guarantee, expressed or implied, that by following the advice below you will make any money or improve current profits, as there are several factors and variables that come into play regarding any given business.

Primarily, results will depend on the nature of the product or business model, the conditions of the marketplace, the experience of the individual, and situations and elements that are beyond your control.

As with any business endeavor, you assume all risk related to investment and money based on your own discretion and at your own potential expense.

Liability Disclaimer

By reading this book, you assume all risks associated with using the advice given below, with a full understanding that you, solely, are responsible for anything that may occur as a result of putting this information into action in any way, and regardless of your interpretation of the advice.

You further agree that our company cannot be held responsible in any way for the success or failure of your business as a result of the information presented in this book. It is your responsibility to conduct your own due diligence regarding the safe and successful operation of your business if you intend to apply any of our information in any way to your business operations.

Terms of Use

You are given a non-transferable, "personal use" license to this book. You cannot distribute it or share it with other individuals.

Also, there are no resale rights or private label rights granted when purchasing this book. In other words, it's for your own personal use only.

Essential Oils & Aromatherapy 101

Top Beauty Secrets for Your Health

By Katie Lenhart

Table of Contents

Introduction

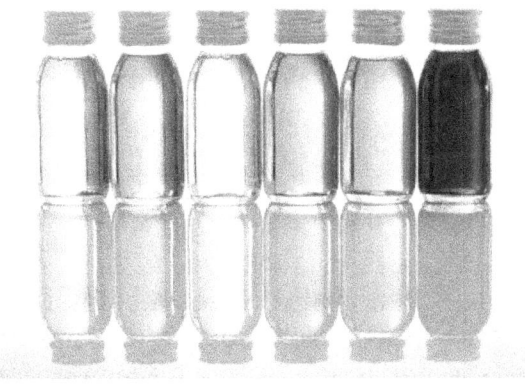

"Essential Oils are your vehicle to strengthened overall health by positively influencing you mind, body and soul. Understanding the basics of these precious yet powerful oils will arm you to fight for great health eternal. Your best move is to make the time to open your mind and learn."

Chemically speaking essential oils consist of teeny molecules much smaller and thus more powerful than molecules found in oils, peanut or sunflower oil for example.

Advantages of small molecules are:

* Increases aromatic abilities, molecules vaporize faster and are absorbed faster.
* This simplifies transferring across cell barriers, inclusive of the blood-brain relationship which instantaneously affects all parts of the body.

* Allows the essential oil molecules to become transdermal, infiltrating the skin quickly and travelling at lightning speed to all parts of your body. For example, you can place some peppermint essential oil on the bottom of your foot and taste it in seconds. Pretty cool, don't you think?

Studies have shown that essential oils help stimulate your immune system and provide support for that ultimate functional balance we strive for to attain optimal health. These volatile essential oils can attack and kill harmful bacteria and viruses, fungus and molds. The antioxidant potential essential oils possess is amazing and powerful. Antioxidants help protect your internal systems for free radical invasion with the sole purpose of initiating serious disease and triggering your eventual demise. Not a pleasant thought, but it is reality.

These volatiles essential oils of nature also influence your mood positively and assist in attaining emotional stability. More commonly, these essential oils are used to revitalize skin and hair, strengthen nails and improve quality sleep, boosting libido, clearing up minor ailments from headaches to joint pain and even influencing improved circulation and absorption of nutrients.

Essential oils are so powerfully potent because they are extremely concentrated. Just a few drops are normally more than enough to trigger a response. To give you an idea, just one single solitary drop of pure peppermint essential oil is equal to almost 30 cups of peppermint tea! That's a heck of a lot of tea. It does make sense when you factor in that almost a whole peppermint plant is used to get just one essence of peppermint oil.

Understanding the basics of these valuable oils of nature is one more positive piece of information you can use to better yourself mind, body and soul. It's a natural alternative to commercial medicines, health and beauty products and interventions that you can file away and perhaps use for your benefit at some point.

This isn't about flipping your life upside down and going nut-so with "essential oil living." It's just a sensible request to open your mind and consider where these natural essential oils might fit into your life. Truth is, if you learn just one new piece of information that is going to benefit you from this book I've done my job and I thank you.

Essential Oil Basics

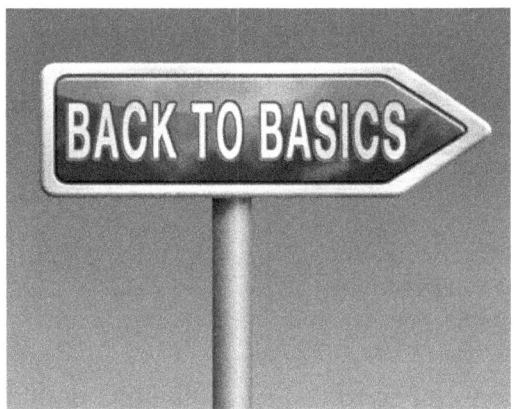

What are essential oils?
Essential oils are simply volatile oils that naturally occur in plants. These oils normally give the plants specific flavors, odors and various other identifiable properties.

They can't ever go bad and are chemically complex. Noting also, they are different than say corn oil because they won't clog pores or leave a greasy feeling. Each of these essential oils is found in various sections of the plant; seeds, stem, flower, bark, often concentrated in one specific location. Just think of the calming scent or vanilla or lavender here.

Some of the uses for essential oils are medicinal, for perfumes and colognes and also flavorings for food products.

Looking into their chemical nature they all vary greatly as one might expect. Most essential oils are made up of carbon and hydrogen and called terpenes. Some consist of phenois or aldehydes and keytones. Various essential oils have the presence of nitrogen, sulfur and oxygen. Bottom line is essential oils are rather complex in nature and we don't need to venture very deep in that.

How to you extract these oils from the plant?

Various methods are used, common ones include:
* distillation by steam
* compression
* pressure
* maceration
* extracting or dissolving oils
* absorbing the oils

A few of the most common essential oils plants are:
* Ginger - cardamom
* Carrot - angelica, anise
* Laurel - camphor
* Heath - wintergreen
* Myrtle - eucalyptus, clove
* Mint - thyme, peppermint, spearmint, pennyroyal
* Rose - almond
* Orchid - vanilla
* Olive - lilac and jasmine
* Pulse - sweet pea, acacia
* Rue - lemon, various citrus plants

FACT - It's the distillation process that makes essential oils so concentrated.

You may also recognize essential oils are ethereal oils, volatile oils or aetherolea. These special oils have been used as medicine for as far back as the history books venture. Medical purposes of these essential oils include:

- skin treatment

14

- cancer treatment

Unfortunately, most of these claims are up for specula-
tion because "science" gets into the equation and it's all
about black and white as you know. Essential oils for
medicinal means is a holistic option for treatment and is
very subjective in nature. It's a tough pill for contempo-
rary medicine to swallow. This doesn't mean these oils
aren't affective or suited to help treat any of these claims.
Point is you will get resistance from the medical society
today. A debate isn't going to happen in this introductory
book!

My Thoughts . . .
Essential oils are a whole lot more than something that
has a nice aroma. They can be used to help improve
your mood, health and thinking or mindset. Up next, we'll
have a look deeper into a few of the more popular essen-
tial oils and uncover the hidden secrets within. Sounds
exciting, don't you think?

Function of Essential Oils in Plants

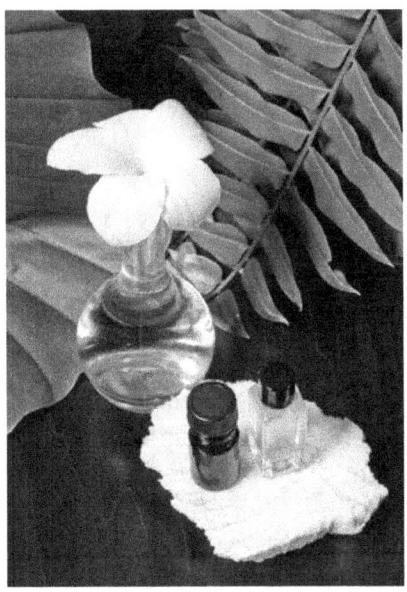

As you know, plants are living things that grow. This process is called assimilation and is executed through oxygen reactions which provide the energy required. There are various substances within the plant always growing and transforming, triggering metabolic reactions and constant change within the plant itself.

The function and creation of flavones, alkaloids and essential oils for example are more difficult to follow. Essential oils are the odor or organic material that plants emit, from the inside out. There are also concentrated amounts of essential oils throughout the plant itself that aren't released as "aroma." Fact is these essential oils are NOT energy sources for plant. Expert researchers know this because even if a plant drops its leaves there are essential oils that remain behind.

From a biological perspective, without getting in too deep, the carbohydrate or starch stores that were in the leaves will step backwards and actually filtrate into the stem of the plant.

So what's the function of essential oils in a plant?

There are a few logical expectations here. The first is these oils create an alluring or attractive sent deemed by nature and the evolution of life itself, to draw in specific insects and animals for the pollination process. In other words, these biological scents produced by the plants are actually manufactured in nature or programmed to attract and repel certain insects and animals, otherwise the eco-system couldn't function productively as it does.

Some experts believe these volatile essential oils serve to act as a means of reserving energy, helping to heal wounds, ward off disease and ensure water is not lost and the plant stays hydrated.

Scientific evidence also shows these oils are "waste" or products of the metabolic process. It is difficult to believe that these powerful and beneficial oils are waste products, which leaves many questioning this reasoning for function. The heat and cooling system of the plant may also be leveled or controlled by essential oils. There are specific oils that help keep to prevent the plant from getting too hot and sweating, just not in large enough quantities to stand strong in theory.

Essential oils can also be harmful and this pushes experts toward validifying the theory these oils really are waste products of the plant. However, if this is the case

it's a blessing in disguise because as you've already be-
gun to see the health benefits of many essential oils
when used safely are fantastic.

My Thoughts . . .
If only plants could talk the scientific community would be
a heck of a lot happier here. With no "black and white"
answers here, experts are forced to observe, experiment
and study these plants in their natural environment and
outside of it in order to fit the pieces of the puzzle togeth-
er as to the true function of essential oils to the plant.
It could very well be they have two or three different func-
tions. It makes sense that they:

* Keep the plant hydrated
* Help heal and keep the plant healthy and resistant to
disease
* Are simply waste products that happen to be hugely
beneficial to humans
It's definitely something to think about and learn from
while understanding more about essential oils in their en-
vironment and more importantly their role with human
health.

10 Popular Essential Oils

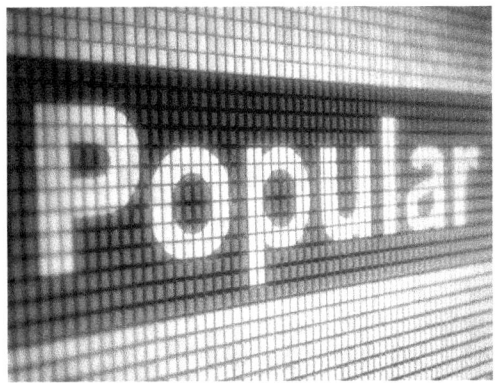

Essential oils are used simply for pure enjoyment of the wonderful scents to treating and preventing health conditions. These are a few of the more common essential oils you might be familiar with.

Eucalyptus - Antiseptic

Most often used to help battle cough, colds and respiratory infections. It's also useful to relieve tense muscles and muscle pain.

Chamomile - Calming

It's used commonly to reduce premenstrual pain and indigestions. Other uses are skin conditions including eczema and acne.

Geranium - Mild Astringent

Very useful for treating mild sores, cuts and fungal infections. Some use it as an effective insect repellant, milk skin problems, bruises and even as an anti-depressant.

Marjoram - Mildly Analgesic

Marjoram is often used to help minimize symptoms of menstruation, headache pain, sore throat and acne. It's also a mild sedative, used to deal with insomnia and even betters circulatory issues.

Rosemary - Mild Stimulant

This essential oil helps alleviate mental and physical tiredness, mild memory loss, asthma and other breathing issues and joint aches and pains.

Sandalwood - Antiseptic

Often used for skin issues such as chapping, dryness or cracked. Also an aphrodisiac and helps with calming during mediation and other relaxation sessions.

Neroli - Mildly Sedative

This volatile oil helps with insomnia, nervousness, anxiety, depression and backache. It's also used for bettering circulation because of its warming qualities.

Jasmine - Anti-depressant

This oil is often used to battle depression, help labor advance and as an aphrodisiac.

Rose - Antiseptic

Sinus issues are often where Rose essential oil is used. It also helps with insomnia, menopause and increases libido.

More Popular Essential oils . . .

Bergamot - Relaxant

This essential oil is orangey smelling and originally from Southeast Asia. It's found in perfumes and colognes and often used to treat emotional issues like stress, depression and anxiety. It can stimulate the liver and improve the function of the digestive system, treat skin infections and boost your mode mildly.

Peppermint - Increases Mental Sharpness

This essential oil is used to bring the skip back into your step. It's also a cooling agent, betters focus, reduces redness and irritation and helps reduce sinus issues.

Lavender - Stress Reducer

Lavender is extremely popular in part to its' relaxing and magnetic scent. It helps to relieve stress, heal and battle head pain, colds and flu effectively. Medicinally, it's used as an anti-inflammatory, antiseptic, antidepressant, diuretic and sedative. Before bed a whiff of lavender will help with relaxation for sleep.

My Thoughts . . .
These are some of the more popular essential oils available. You can see that each has unique qualities and uses. These oils are holistic natural methods of dealing with the inevitable aches and pains that come with life.

Uses of Essential Oils

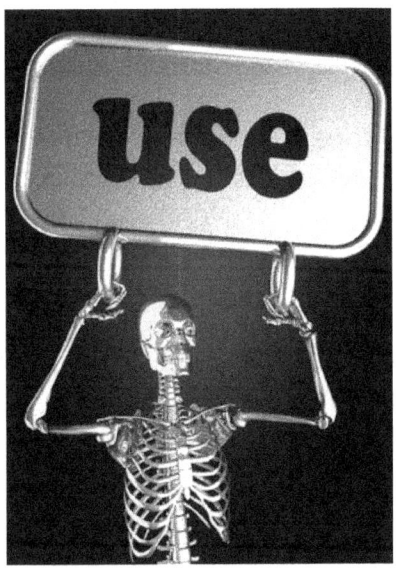

Essential oils are growing in popularity as people are making the shift from absolute conventional thinking into more natural and non-invasive means of living, opting for choices less detrimental to the environment and more "gentle" in nature to begin with.

These oils are all natural, found in nature and experts have uncovered numerous purposeful uses for each. Of course you add a magnetic fragrance to your home, at least that's what many associate essential oils with. Though attention is now being shifted to the invaluable and often unknown benefits due to the therapeutic nature of these oils.

These volatile and powerful "essences of nature" are a gynormous part of natural and holistic medicine, healing and living. Keep in mind these oils are extremely concentrated and caution must be exercised at all times. Too much of anything in life isn't a good thing. A little goes a long way here with a drop or two often being plenty. Some of the uses for essential oils are:

* Salt Scrub - Peppermint works well here. You just mix one cup of salt with approximately 1/2 cup olive or grape seed oil and add about 10 drops of essential oil. This is an excellent for naturally exfoliating the skin and leaving it baby bottom soft.

* Lip Balm - Essential oils work wonderful for creating moisture for your lips.

RECIPE:
1 tablespoon beeswax pearls
1/8 cup coconut oil
1/2 tablespoon shea butter
1/2 tablespoon cocoa butter
3/4 teaspoon honey
Liquid from 2-3 vitamin E gel capsules
1 teaspoon cocoa powder
3 drops of your favorite essential oil

Put the two butters in a small pot and heat on low for about 15 minutes stirring intermittently. Toss in the beeswax and blend well to melt. Take the mixture off the heat and add your favorite essential oil, vitamin E, honey and cocoa powder stirring continuously. Place in lip balm container and leave it to set about 2 hours.

* Skin Oil Moisturizer - Combine 1 cup of olive or grape seed oil with about 60 drops of your favorite essential oil.

This is fabulous as a natural moisturizer in or after your bath or shower.

* Natural Deodorant - The essential oils help to kill bacteria and keep odor away, along with preventing perspiration.
* Toothpaste - Bet you never thought of this one! Essential oils are great for making your own toothpaste. You just need coconut oil, baking soda and peppermint essential oil.
* Zit Zapper - Tee tree essential oil works wonderfully on stopping a pimple in its tracks, reducing redness and drying it up.
* Mouthwash - Believe it or not peppermint, wintergreen or spearmint oils make a fabulous mouthwash.
* Air Freshener - Add your favorite essential oil to baking soda and you've just made air freshener. Pour baking soda into a glass jar until half full. Add about 20 drops of essential oil, poke holes in the top and shake!
* Household Cleaner - Just add a few drops of essential oil to white vinegar for a environmentally friendly cleaner that works.
* Vapor Spray - Add about 20 drops of essential oil to a spray bottle filled with distilled water and you've got a natural odor-eating spray.
* Laundry Scent - Add your favorite essential oil to your laundry detergent to give it a pleasant scent.
* Deodorize Mattress - Take a cup of baking soda and add approximately 20 drops of lavender or your favorite oil. Sprinkle on mattress and leave for a few hours. Vacuum up and you've got a clean mattress.
* Sunburn Relief - Add about 20 drops lavender to two cups water in spray bottle and "spritz" on sunburn for relief.
* Itching - Add 10 drops lavender oil to base oil and apply liberally to insect bite or itch.

* Cold Sores - Applying tea tree essential oil directly will help heal.
* Headache/Migraine/TMJ relief - Use peppermint essential oil directly on forehead, neck and temples to battle your head pain.
* Massage Oils - Picking your favorite essential oil and using as a lubricant to massage is simply fabulous. Lavender is very relaxing and smells like heaven.

There are just so many uses for essential oils that if you put your mind to it I bet you can come up with a few new ones on your own. Essential oils are all good in the game of life when looking to better your health, mind, body and soul.

My Thoughts . . .
There are so many uses for these powerfully beneficial essential oils that it's hard to keep track. You now have a good understanding of various uses for the more common oils out there. Step by step you can implement these practical uses into your beauty regimen to improve your complexion, reduce stress, alleviate annoying aches and pains and even battle serious disease. The sky is the limit with essential oils and your great health. Open your mind and spread your wings with this opportunity to soar.

Health Benefits

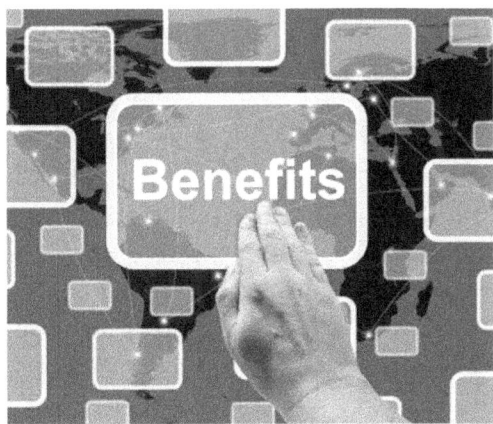

Essential oils should have their place in your daily beauty regimen. These oils are all-natural, free of added chemicals or modifications and can be used for anything from cleaning to beauty products and even health means. These oils are up to one-hundred times more powerful than herbs and this means more effectiveness in their purpose.

Throughout history essential oils have been used for all sorts of health issues. Experts aren't saying they are the end-all-be-all for good health, although they will stand by the fact they can make your health better, having been used to deal with digestions issues and acne, to battling serious germs and so forth.

Here are a few essential oils that pack power in their punch.

Geranium

Holistic specialists suggest adding geranium oil to your PMS fighting ritual to help reduce symptoms. It doesn't stop here though because it's also used to reduce redness and inflammation on the skin. It's typically great for battling acne and those oil skin cycles reflective of hormone changes.

Peppermint

Peppermint not only soothes or rather tames bad breath, it also works to alleviate nausea and various other stomach issues, stop itching and relax overworked muscles. If you are congested just add a few drops of peppermint to steaming water and breathe in. Peppermint also helps battle symptoms of PMS, soothe sore throats and cough and get rid of pesky headaches.

Lavender

This essential oil seems to be the "go-to" of oils. Spas in particular use lavender oil for just about everything. It is very gentle and can essentially be used straight up. This oil fights germs, aids digestion, helps alleviate head pain, calms and relaxes, improves sleep, reduces joint and muscle pain, clear urinary tract infections, lowers blood pressure, zaps acne and even helps with respiratory issues. Wow!

Sesame

Hair and skin treatments tend to use sesame essential oil. The fatty acids in this oil are believed to help lower stress, blood pressure and even retard the growth of cancer cells. Studies show sesame essential oil even has a touch of SPF factor. Sounds great to me!

Rose

This specialty oil is often noted and used for its alluring and relaxing aroma. Beyond this it also helps with leveling hormones, reducing blood pressure, lessening meno-menopausal symptoms, improving complexion and boosting performance in the bedroom.

Here are some more benefits of these volatile oils with so much power.

* Boosts Stamina and Memory - Try a glass of water with 3-4 drops of lemon, orange or peppermint oil added.
* Sleep Issues - To help with insomnia just add a few drops of lavender oil onto a cloth and place under your pillow.
* Strengthen Immune System - After bathing put a few drops of thyme or oregano oil to the bottom of your feet.
* Deter Motion Sickness - Put a few drops of peppermint oil on a towel and breathe in periodically during the trip.
* Battles Bacteria and Fungus - Essential oils added to an air mist device or diffuser will help protect against nasty microbes.

Technical Benefits of Administering, Breathing or Diffusing Pure Essential Oils

- More oxygen to the cell
- Increased efficiency in production and reception of Human Growth Hormone
- Higher secretions of "feel good" chemicals or endorphins
- More production of ATP which is energy used by cells
- Increased efficiency in removing and utilizing protein from amino acids
- Antibodies are manufactured faster which helps hinder disease
- More serotonin and hormone release

- Faster healing because histamines are released in greater quantities
- Improved circulation and strengthened immunity
- Ability to better handle emotional turmoil
- Increased chemical production overall to heighten bodily function efficiency

My Thoughts . . .
Healing of the mind and body with essential oils has been used for centuries, treating a wide array of surface and internal issues naturally. Every oil has a distinct scent, flavor and purpose and for the most part is used separately. These oils have been studied deeply and are used safely and effectively to better your health. Knowledge is power and the aim of this book is to give you some new practical knowledge you can apply for better health and happiness.

Caution

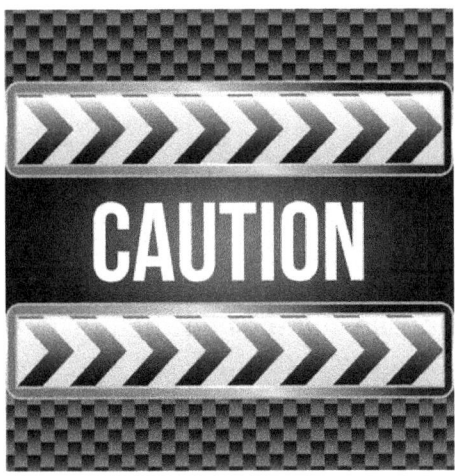

Hands down the most dangerous aspect of essential oils is the belief that because they are natural they can't ever be harmful.

ESSENTIAL OILS CAN BE FATAL IF USED IN LARGE QUANTITIES!

Truth is there are lots of different toxins present in nature. Just keep this in mind when you are picking your essential oils to use and ensure you know what levels are safe. Don't run scared here just make sure you use common sense and caution.

Unwise Use

The majority of essential oils need to be watered down or diluted for topical application. This is because they are so concentrated naturally. If you don't dilute an oil properly, it may even burn your skin. Make sure you never add a little extra essential like you might add gin to your drink. Just don't do it and you've got nothing to worry about. If you are using essential oils with aromatherapy and increase the concentration this can cause vomiting or headaches. It's just not something you want to have to deal with.

Skin Issues

Some people just naturally have sensitive skin regardless of the product applied. When trying an essential oil out on your skin you're best to test it first to ensure you won't react. Just because something is natural doesn't mean your body is going to accept it.

Take note some essential oils are not appropriate for skin use.

Pet Cautions

Tea tree oil might very well trigger vomiting, weakness and nausea in dogs. Cats are even more sensitive to the powerful medicinal qualities in essential oils so proceed with caution and make certain you have the correct knowledge before applying. The liver of a cat isn't physiologically able to handle the toxins in these oils according to experts.

Birds are more sensitive than cats and even inhaling a whiff of an essential oil can kill them. Just picture precious little "tweetie bird" here.

General Dangers

The majority of essential oils are not made to eat. Unless you have qualified information from a medical professional you should NEVER ingest essential oils just to be safe. The oils are highly concentrated and may be toxic to your system.

These oils are also easily absorbed into the skin which makes them more dangerous to a pregnant woman or a couple trying to get pregnant.

My Thoughts . . .

Common sense goes a long way here in avoiding trouble. If you are unsure of how to use a specific essential oil, do yourself a favor and don't until you are sure. These oils can be extremely beneficial to your health, but they aren't going to be of use to you if you act irresponsibly. This is not a lecture, it's just wise a fact.

Essential Oils and Weight Loss

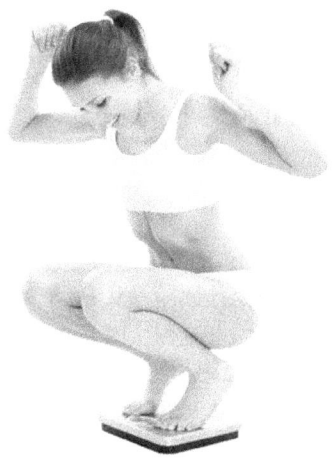

Health and wellness experts agree that pure and natural essential oils including bergamot, grapefruit, peppermint and sandalwood will help accelerate weight loss when combined with healthy eating and regularly exercise. It's a piece of the big picture that will only get you healthier faster.

Of course there are no guarantees in life, but weight loss is most definitely linked with these essential oils in particular. As well, they will boost mood, increase energy levels, and flip your life switch to positive, making your day more invigorating and exciting. Here are a few herbs for weight loss that are worth your attention.

Bergamot

Experts agree bergamot helps level emotional stress and anxiety which often causes overeating. Your endocrine system works with bergamot to instill calm and deter or minimize stress. By also using lavender essential oil you will only heighten the effects.

You can also place a few drops of bergamot on a cloth and inhale to relax. Using bergamot in your daily routine is beneficial in weight loss.

Grapefruit

This volatile oil helps dissolve fat and eliminate bloating naturally. Limonene is an ingredient found in grapefruit essential oil that assists in releasing heart healthy fatty acids into the bloodstream. They are broken down and utilized for energy. Studies show this essential oil also acts to suppress hunger, which is ideal when trying to lose weight. Placing a few drops on a cloth and inhaling works wonders for many.

Peppermint

This essential oil is interesting as it has the ability to interfere with the chemical message sent from the hypothalamus in the brain or control center, that you are hungry. Peppermint alters the message to tell the brain you're full. It also aids naturally in digestion and can alleviate tummy troubles.

Benefits and achieved by placing a few drops of peppermint essential oil on a towel and inhaling or a few drops in your water before eating.

Sandalwood

This essential oil provides a natural "feel-good" feeling. It acts as a sedative, treatment for mild skin conditions and cleans skin. Researchers have also found it can alter the behavior of negative cell intentions and actions. Sandalwood has the ability to tell the brain "moderation," which helps encourage less food and a better chance for losing weight. Self-confidence and self control is huge in weight loss success and this essential oil delivers both. Your mind is a powerful thing and to feel calm and completely in control of your actions and thoughts is only going to help you with losing weight.

Some herbs specialists have identified that help cellulite are:

* rosemary, thyme, allspice, cumin, cypress, lavender, lemon, pine
* sage, tangerine, lime, oregano, sweet fennel, landalin, sweet basil, cinnamon leaf
* sassafras, storax, lovage, orange, fir needle, grapefruit, geranium, bay, celery seed
* bezoin, sweet birch, cassia bark

Brain Chemistry and Weight Loss

You have the physical action plan for weight loss which includes watching portion sizes, eating a wide variety of healthy foods and exercising. Now researchers are looking into brain chemistry and how essential oils can alter the amount of food you eat and the desire for it. This of course, can help you lose weight.

What essential oils can do is to increase your feeling of self-satisfaction and boost low self confidence. These specialty oils can also control and get rid of cellulite. The learned response for eating is:

to see the food, smell the food and want it, then eat it
What if the response was:
to see the food, smell the food and NOT want it, then NOT eat it

Explanation

Many people believe hunger is triggered by low blood sugar levels, what has been discovered is a part in the brain known as the nucleus of the hypothalamus that controls your "feeling full" message.

By intercepting and altering the hypothalamus we can reduce eating. Scientists know that your nose is connected and can be used change the hunger message to your brain by smelling essential oils that deter hunger. Scientists believe scents that deter hunger are peppermint, banana and green apple.

Metabolism and Weight Loss

Studies have long since show herbs including thyme, pink grapefruit, lime, lemon, orange, basil, rosemary, spearmint and peppermint encourage weight loss. Researchers now know that smelling these essential oils triggers the same affect.

In theory, you can use these essential oils to help with weight management my inhaling them deeply. This must be done directly from the bottle with one nostril closed for full effect. Slow deep breathes need to be taken repeatedly a few times a day, ensuring you use different oils is important because this will satiate the body for different foods.

Lemon and grapefruit essential oils are used specifically to increase metabolism and aid in weight loss. You can make these oils into perfumes to place on your body and inhale by combining up to 10 drops of oil with 2-3 teaspoons sweet almond oil.

Essential oils to add to bath or massage for weight loss are:
- Sage, thyme or basil essential oils
- Lavender, spearmint or lemon essential oils
- Rosemary, lime or pink grapefruit essential oils
- Melissa, oregano, peppermint or orange essential oils
Essential oils used to treat obesity are:
- Orange, lemon, lime and pink grapefruit essential oils

My Thoughts . . .
To each his/her own. Even qualified experts debate back and forth which essential oils best promotes weight loss. Troubles arise in the fact it's not just one factor that determines if your body is going to purge fat and how quickly. Does a relaxed body better metabolize fat? Is it more beneficial to get less sleep and exercise more or vice versa to increase your metabolism to lose weight faster? Does your body absorb and use pink grapefruit or lemon more effectively? You can see each of these factors is but impossible to measure accurately simply because we all are uniquely different structurally and mentally. As with most efforts of change the mind needs to be open to some experimenting and figuring out what works best for you, which essential oils and in what amounts, combined with healthy eating and regular exercise will help you blast fat the fastest and keep it off. Time for you to get started don't you think?

Feature Alzheimer's and Essential Oil Hope

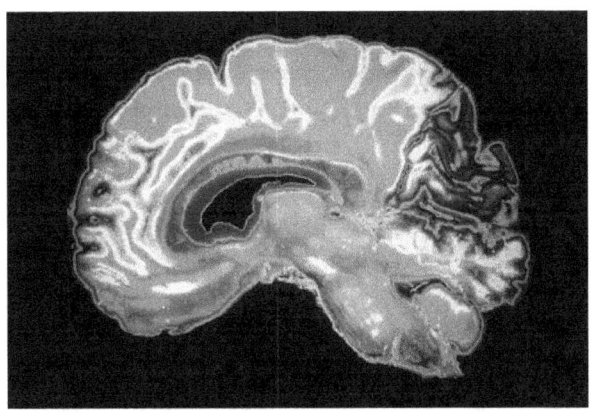

Alzheimer's is basically a degenerative disease of the brain that's progressive in nature, where thinking, cognitive execution and memory become interfered with. Alzheimer's is the main form of dementia according to the medical community.

What is dementia?

A syndrome or condition where various functions of the brain are impaired. The inability to think clearly, recall memories, make logical judgments, extreme moods flips and being unable to communicate clearly are all common observations with dementia.

Research shows essential oils help improve:
* cognitive capacity
* agitation issue
* behavior

43

* memory
* aggressive nature
* mood
* memory recall

Rosemary, peppermint and lemon essential oils aid with improved memory and awareness.

Ylang-ylang, lavender and orange help calm, sedate and lift depression. For sleep issues, lavender and mandarin are recommended.

Research shows those suffering from Alzheimer's also have an issue with smelling or they have a dysfunction related to their olfactory. The good news is that essential oils don't have to be inhaled because they are most affective on a physiological platform. These volatile oils actually infiltrate the body via the lungs and skin tissue. Seeing as the chemical makeup of these essential oils is concentrated and complex, they are effective. Think of it as drinking an orange drink that has 10% real juice versus eating a REAL orange. It is a huge difference in nutritional value and health benefits.

Bottom line is extensive research shows lavender essential oil is most beneficial for Alzheimer's treatment if you had to choose just one. A simple massage of the hand with pure lavender helps positive emotion, deterring aggressiveness which is detrimental and very difficult to deal with.

Another common combination to help lift cognitive function is lavender and orange in the early evening and lemon and rosemary essential oils throughout the day. The great new is there are no side effects reported. Of course with conventional medicinal treatment options the side effects are just the beginning of issues triggered.

Thyme essential oil is also significant in the treatment and management of Alzheimer's because it targets AChE specifically which is an enzyme that degrades acetylcholine, a neurotransmitter.

Add to this the fact studies have shown sage essential oil has the ability to lift your mood and increase the rate in which you recall memories. Research and complex experimentation has also divulged lemon balm essential oil aids in decreasing agitation which is a common symptom of interference in Alzheimer's patients.

My Thoughts . . .
Bottom line is when your back is against the wall and there's so much unknown with Alzheimer's, having the option of a natural treatment option is very inviting. Again it's all about trial and error because no two people are the same. Using effective essential oils to assist in handling, stress, fear, anxiety, confusion, depression, aggression and panic attacks, all associated with Alzheimer's is a move worthy of serious consideration.

Simple Beauty and Skincare Tips

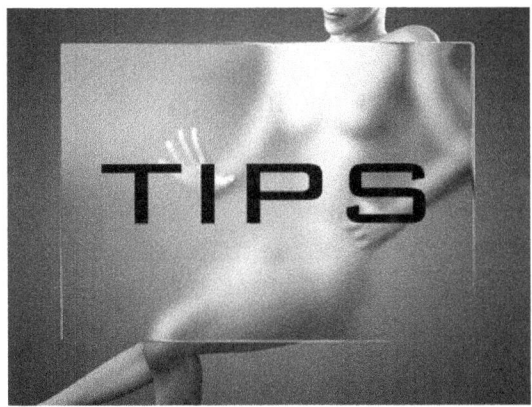

Essential oils can be fabulous for restoring and maintaining skin and are often a part of skin care regimens.

Lavender Oil Beauty Tips

* By adding about five drops of this essential oil to a glass of milk you can make a luxurious skin softening agent for your bath.
* Lavender oil kills lice and helps with hair growth when massaged into the scalp.
* Adding this oil to jojoba oil and slipping into your bath will help soothe painful sunburn.

Tea-Tree Oil

* You can add a few drops of this essential oil to some yogurt and apply it to your skin to alleviate oily skin.
* Nail fungus doesn't stand a chance with a few drops of tea-tree oil.

* By adding some of this volatile oil to your shampoo and massaging it into your scalp you will help moisturize and strengthen your hair.

Rosemary Oil

* Stimulates hair follicles so hair grows in thicker and stronger while moisturizing the scalp naturally.
Rosewood Oil

* Spraying this essential oil mixed with hot water on an absorbent towel then wrap around yourself. Cover with blanket and feel the toxins leave through your skin.

Mandarin or Lemon Oil

* To get rid of dark circles under eyes put a couple drops of oil into a bowl of hot water, place a towel over your head and "tent" to steam onto your face.

Au Natural Body Lotion

Use about 6 ounces non-scented organic lotion and add 12 drops myrrh, 12 drops geranium and about 3 drops ylang-ylang essential oils. This works wonders lathering on after a relaxing bath.

Nail Strengthener

Start with 2-3 tablespoons of pure vitamin E oil. Mix in 10 drops each of lemon, myrrh and frankincense essential oils and apply a few times a week to cuticles.

Gentle Skin Toner

Start with 6-8 ounces pure water. Add 2 drops lavender oil, 1 drop palmarosa and rosewood essential oils. Place in a bottle, shake and apply with cotton ball.

My Thinking . . .
Essential oils are excellent candidates to freshen up your beauty routine. These fabulously fragrant oils from nature will help maintain your youthful appearance and battle the harmful effects of our harsh environment and often stressful lifestyles.
You never know unless you step outside your comfort zone and give it a try right?

Fact or Fiction?

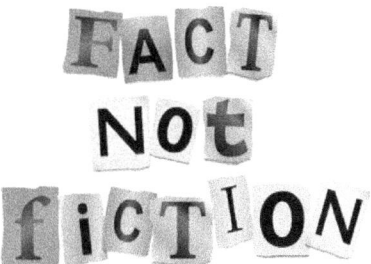

Sometimes sorting fact from fiction is downright annoying! In general, the simpler and more straight forward the information, the more likely it is going to be accurate fact. If your gut is telling your something is a little quirky about the words you are pondering don't be afraid to question its validity. Usually your natural instincts are correct. The problem with misinformation is often as simple as learning not to trust yourself, to always second guess and then it's next to impossible to sort through to the true of the matter.

Here are a few "fictions" turned fact to help you rest your brain and absorb the base and accurate information you need to build on your essential oil knowledge.

Fiction 1 - There is only one place or company you can get REAL essential oils from, the rest are just fakes.

Fact: I don't know who started this one except maybe the supposed one and only supplier of essential oils to the whole freaking world! Come on people. There are lots of valid companies around the globe taking the time to manufacture volatile essential oils in the purest form.

Now this industry isn't regulated as closely as many would like so it's important to do your research BEFORE buying just to ensure you are getting what you're paying for. Understanding essential oils aren't cheap by any means, but they do go a long way.

One key concern is if an essential oil isn't distilled properly it will not be as effective when it's time to step up to the plate. Figure out who you know and who you trust and don't forget to follow your gut.

Fiction 2 - Essential oils are all-mighty powerful. The ultimate energies of the plant kingdom hold the key to life as we speak. Perhaps we should bow down now?

Fact: Don't mean to burst your bubble, but you aren't going to make friends with essential oils anytime soon because they aren't living. Would you be alive if you went through a distillation process at over 200 degrees? I think not!

These essential oils are simply a combination of volatile dead molecules and therefore give nothing to life. When it comes to the actual making of essential oils, plants do so at different times during their development. Essential oils are really the end or near end result of plant metabolism.

Fiction 3 - Volatile essential oils are made of macro and micronutrients, proteins, carbohydrates, fats, vitamins and minerals.

Fact: What the heck are you talking about here? Never mind all those elements above. Essential oils are made of oxygen, carbon and hydrogen. They are sensitive organic liquids with no hormones, vitamins or minerals.

Fiction 4 - A rash or burn mark from an essential oil is just part of the detoxification process.

Fact: Just like picking a hot pan out of the oven and burning the crap out of your hands is good for practicing healing. Let it be time to think logically here. If you happen to rub a wild plant of sorts on your skin and break out in a rash, is that called detoxification? Obviously it isn't and if you are getting a rash or any other sort of skin irritation from essential oils than you it's irritating your skin for some reason and you need to do something about it. With essential oils it's usually because the concentration is too high and you either need to mix it with something or use less. When your body reacts like that it's telling you to stop and reassess. Do yourself a favor and listen, please!

Fiction 5 - If you want "better" or "faster" results just use a little more essential oil. This saves you time.

Fact: NO, NO, NO! Essential oils are not like a bag of cookies. If you are looking to get fat faster, just eat more. These oils are extremely dangerous when used stupidly. Make sure you use the proper "drop" ratios always and if you are unsure ask a reliable source. If your instructions are to use 5 drops don't think 10 drops will get you faster results. Bottom line is essential oils can be toxic when misused.

Think here and be safe and you'll have nothing to lose and everything to gain.

Fiction 6 - The first pressing of an essential oil is the best!

Fact: Not true whatsoever and who said anything about pressing? Are we talking about essential oils or apples? For the most part essential oils are derived from a steam distillation process. Citrus oils are cold pressed but that's got nothing to do with "first pressing" and best quality.

These precious plants are never steam distilled more than once. It's not like cutting hay from a field where you get first, second and usual a third cut. Where the third cut usually yields less and doesn't have the quality and texture of the first cut. Pure essential oils are pure essential oils, a one shot deal. So you don't have to worry about second and third takes here because that just doesn't happen.

Fiction 7 - Essential oils will cure just about everything fast.

Fact: It won't take you long to figure out essential oils are not the ultimate cure for everything. What they do is offer viable natural holistic options for treating health issues and ailments. They look to promote good health and work best in combination with healthy eating, exercising and mental health. Find the parts that work with essential oils and fit them into your life.

Fiction 8 - You need to study essential oils for quite some time before you are going to benefit from them.

Fact: This one just isn't true. The truth is volatile essential oils are easy to use. By taking a few minutes to learn which essential oil you are using, why and how much you need, you will do just fine. The last thing you want to do is complicate things here. Essential oils are safe and effective and honestly really easy to use. Don't let this fallacy mess up your thinking and send you running.

Fiction 9 - Using essential oils will make you healthy without bothering with anything else.

Fact: You can't give up our healthy lifestyle and expect essential oil to pick up the slack.

Fiction 10 - Only those people that shun conventional medicine use essential oils only.

Fact: Truth is many who use conventional medicine use essential oils and many who practice holistic medicine also use conventional methods of treatment when warranted. Most often people use essential oils to add to or compliment their chosen treatment regimen. That makes the most sense, don't you think?

Fiction 11 - If are pregnant, elderly or have children, essential oils should never be used.

Fact: There are always exceptions to the rules. Yes, there are some essential oils that shouldn't be used when pregnant or on children and they are clearly labeled so. An example is that lavender has been known to trigger premature labor. Just proceed with the same caution you would when taking a medication.

Simply ensure you understand what essential oil you are taking and why. Also triple check to ensure it's safe for your situation. Be smart and always put safety first!

Fiction 12 - Essential oils will break the bank.

Fact: This one depends on perception. There are some essential oils that are quite expensive but you have to consider the fact that very little is required for full effect. It's up to decide if you think essential oils are worth the money or not. To me and many others they really are worth their weight in gold.

Fiction 13 - You can ingest essential oils for full affect.

Fact: This myth is very wrong. Rule 101 here is these oils are not made for ingestion period. The only exception to the rule here is if you were working closely with a qualified specialist you trust and have been instructed otherwise. Then I would re-check the terms and conditions of your life insurance policy before proceeding, just to confirm the beneficiary.

My Thoughts . . .
As you can read there are lots of myths out there about essential oils and we've just taken the first bite here. Bottom line is it's very important to have accurate information when you're looking to make changes to better your health. Doesn't matter if it's habit changes in eating or exercising or looking for alternative natural methods to treat chronic or annoying conditions. Beginning with the facts is going to steer you straighter that slip sliding through half-truths.
Hope these truths give you a piece of mind and arm you with the positive and practical information you need to make awesome decisions towards great health.

Final Thoughts

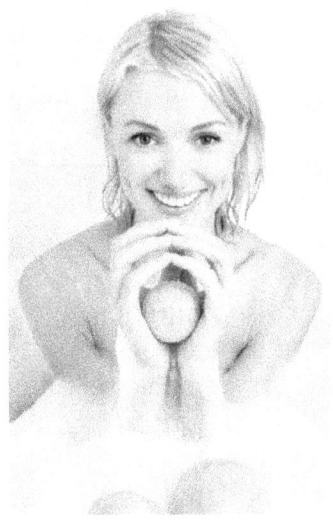

Perhaps is the subtle calming scent of lavender or the sweet drawing aroma of orange that leaves you smiling when sensing these pure and effective essential oils of nature. Bonus is the fact they are often beneficial in bettering your health by speeding up the healing process, strengthening your immune system, clearing up skin conditions and helping to increase circulation and "strengthen" internal systems. There is just so much more to essential oils that you see on the surface.

Essential oils are what you want to suit your purpose of better health, although there are different "kinds" of essential oils that aren't as pure in production that have other purposes. Essential oils can be "tinkered" with in order to change concentration, effectiveness and cost.

This isn't a good or bad thing, just is and as long as you are aware of what you are buying all is well.

The four different grades of essential oils are:

A Grade - These are oils that are pure and natural, used for health therapy and are distilled in a scientific process uninhibited. Highest concentrations are present here.

B Grade - Food grade oils fall here because they often have extenders or extra oils added to lessen the cost and serve an alternate purpose.

C Grade - Essential oils found here are suitable for perfumes and colognes, similar to food grade oils these essential oils usually have solvents and additives that stretch the oils farther. Unfortunately, the additives to these oils are not healthy and pure, but they serve purpose in the perfume industry. This is not surprisingly cost is a major factor here. Just like watering down soda with ice, extending the essential oils is going to drop the cost dramatically and still enable perfume manufacturers to use the label of "essential oils" to sell their product.

Floral Water - This is just the leftovers of the essential oils distillation process. It's high quality water from the distillation process that has quantities of essential oils for use. If a high grade distillation process is used the floral water is very high in quality. Of course if the process isn't top quality, the results will be poor too.

Sure you may get the aroma, smell and "sense" of the powerful essential oil, but the chemical makeup serves weaker and not effective. Think of it as smelling an orange and actually tasting one. If you want the health benefits of an orange you need to eat it. Sure by smelling one you can experience of lead your mind to believe you're experiences all the orange has to offer but in reality you aren't.

Pure and precious essential oils are viewed invaluable, protected and savored by individuals that understand the awesome benefits and powers of essential oils utilized properly and with respect. Nourishing, rejuvenating, regenerating and cleansing thoroughly are just a few functions of essential oils introduced to the human body.

The magic begins just beneath the surface of the skin where an interconnection throughout the whole body is established. Think of this as a layer of flowing water where anything that enters can flow freely throughout the body and benefit where needed. The heart may need some essential oil to relax and work more effectively. This particular oil might skip right past the lungs because they have their eyes peeled for a different oil to benefit from. Do you see where I'm going here?

It's almost impossible for experts to determine and understand all the positive benefits and how they come about with essential oils. There are just too many to name and the processes themselves once these oils enter your system are intricately complex and tough to follow or measure. These oils may be inhaled, absorbed through the skin, soaked with helper substances, allowed in with heat, sometimes your body takes an essential oil in with each absorption method.

Add to this the uniqueness your bodily function and it's fair to say you might absorb and benefit from 5 drops of lavender essential oil differently than I would. Your internal makeup or bodily blueprint might dictate rosemary essential oil is preferred over rose essential oil for no other reason than it's what your system prefers.

Opening your mind to experiment with these incredibly beneficial essential oils of nature will only help strengthen your mind and body. Through direct application, inhalation or on rare occasion internally allowing the essence of nature into your daily regimen is only going to manifest positive health gain . . .

* Increasing energy
* Fighting off disease
* Strengthening cognitive capacity
* Improving physical function
* Removing stress
* Slowing the aging process
* Deterring serious illness and disease
* Firming skin
* Healing minor wounds and ailments
* Preserving life quality
* Flipping your internal switch to positive

Essential oils will open the doors of opportunity that for many have been sealed shut. Are you ready to step through those doors and start benefitting?

We have the choice to look for the positive or the negative in life. You can choose to lift someone up or to stomp on them. Writing is my passion and I work hard at it, with the goal of helping make people better. If you gain a new piece of knowledge, read something that makes you think, or perhaps even smile a few times, then I am happy and content!

Life's just too short not to tune into optimism. If your glass is half full, then I invite you to read my writing, and if you have a minute to spare when you're through, **I would appreciate your review.** This will help me better myself and my writing. I thank you in advance and appreciate you.

www.ingramcontent.com/pod-product-compliance
Lightning Source LLC
Chambersburg PA
CBHW070820290526
45795CB00002B/783